CERVICAL SPONDYLOSIS

How to Avoid and Deal with Cervical Spondylosis: Tips for Long-Term Health

CARL JUAN

Table of Contents

Introductory

Cervical spondylosis is a degenerative disorder of the cervical spine (the top part of the spine, in the neck), often known as cervical osteoarthritis or neck arthritis. It's caused by the natural breakdown of the vertebrae (backbones) and the discs that act as shock absorbers as we become older. Symptoms and problems of this degenerative process include:

• Pain in the neck is a common symptom of cervical spondylosis, and it can vary in intensity from mild to severe.

• Reduced flexibility in the neck can make it painful to turn the head or move it in any direction.

• Caused by neck muscular tension or nerve compression, headaches are a common symptom of cervical spondylosis.

• Compression of the nerves as they leave the cervical spine can cause discomfort to spread from the neck into the shoulders, arms, and even the hands.

• Arm, hand, and finger numbness and weakness are additional symptoms associated with nerve compression.

- Cervical spondylosis has been linked to a decline in fine motor abilities, making it difficult for those affected to do things like button a shirt or handle small objects.

- Compromised bowel or bladder function is a rare but serious complication of cervical spondylosis, which can occur when the spinal cord is compressed. This is a very dangerous symptom that needs to be checked out right away.

Cervical spondylosis is a degenerative disorder that mainly affects people over the age of 40 and worsens over time. Cervical spondylosis can be caused by a variety of factors, including aging, heredity, bad posture, and neck injuries in the past.

Cervical spondylosis treatment varies according on the severity of the condition. Physical therapy, pain management, anti-inflammatory drugs, and lifestyle changes are common components of conservative treatment plans. Surgery to relieve nerve compression or stabilize the spine may be an option in severe cases where non-invasive treatments have failed. Neck discomfort and other symptoms may be signs of cervical spondylosis, so it's crucial to see a doctor if you have any of these concerns.

CHAPTER ONE
Factors and Predisposing Causes

Several prevalent causes and risk factors contribute to the development of cervical spondylosis, but the aging process and the wear and tear on the cervical spine are the primary culprits. Among these are:

• The majority of cases of cervical spondylosis are brought on by the natural aging process. Degeneration of the cervical spine occurs when the spinal discs dry out and become less flexible, and when the vertebrae grow bone spurs.

• Cervical spondylosis may run in families, therefore some people may be predisposed to the condition. There may be a higher chance of developing this ailment if it runs in one's family.

• Accidental or repetitive trauma to the neck, such as that sustained in a vehicle accident or while playing a contact sport, can lead to cervical spondylosis. Degeneration of the cervical spine can be hastened by injury.

• **Repetitive Stress:** Cervical spondylosis can be brought on by long-term mechanical stress and bad posture. Neck injuries are more likely to occur in jobs or hobbies that require constant neck bending or twisting.

• The chance of developing cervical spondylosis is greater in people who smoke. It may disrupt the blood flow to the cervical spine, perhaps increasing deterioration.

• **Occupational Factors:** Certain activities that involve heavy lifting, carrying, or other physical demands on the neck and spine can contribute to the development of cervical spondylosis. Another risk factor is sitting for lengthy periods of time with bad posture.

- Causes of degeneration of the cervical spine include obesity, which places extra strain on the spine.

- Cervical spondylosis is more prevalent in males than females, regardless of age. However, the causes underlying this gender disparity are not entirely understood.

- Cervical spondylosis risk is increased by sedentary lifestyles and failing to engage in regular physical activity. Keeping up with a healthy and active routine can aid in lowering this possibility.

- When using a computer or other electronic device that does not have proper ergonomics, strain can be placed on the neck, which can lead to cervical spondylosis. Ergonomics and a well-organized desk can significantly lessen exposure.

Cervical spondylosis is more likely in those who already have one or more of these risk factors, but this is by no means guaranteed. Cervical spondylosis is a common age-related illness, and mild to moderate degeneration may exist in many persons without causing noticeable symptoms. Consult a medical expert for an assessment and individualized recommendations for prevention and management if you are worried about your risk or if you are experiencing neck discomfort and related symptoms.

Structure and Function of the Cervical Spine

The cervical spine is an important component of the human spine, located in the neck area and consisting of the first seven vertebrae of the vertebral column (C1 to C7). It's crucial because it helps keep the head steady, safeguards the spinal cord, and enables other bodily processes. The structure and function of the cervical spine are summarized below.

Cervical Spine Anatomy:

• Cervical vertebrae are numbered from C1 to C7 and make up the cervical spine. Vertebrae in the cervical spine are more mobile and pliable than those in the thoracic and lumbar regions of the spine.

• **Intervertebral Discs:** Between each pair of cervical vertebrae are intervertebral discs. These discs perform the dual roles of cushioning the neck and allowing for range of motion. The nucleus pulposus is the inner core and the annulus fibrosus is the outer layer of these structures.

•   The spinal cord is a key component of the central nervous system that is encased in and protected by the cervical spine. The spinal cord acts as a conduit for the transmission of both sensory and motor nerve impulses to and from the brain.

•   Foramina are tiny apertures between adjacent cervical vertebrae where nerve roots emerge from the spinal cord. These nerve roots branch out to different regions of the body and regulate sensation and motion there.

• Facet joints, which connect adjacent vertebrae, are just one example of the many joints and ligaments found in the cervical spine. The ligaments in the spine are responsible for its rigidity and strength.

Cervical Spine Role in Body Function:

• The cervical spine's main job is to hold up the head, which weighs about 10 to 12 pounds (4.5 to 5.4 kg) on average. The skull is supported by the first cervical vertebra, or atlas, while the second, or axis, enables the head to move in a pivoting motion.

• Nodding the head up and down, tilting it to the side, and rotating it are only some of the many movements made possible by the cervical spine's pliability. The ability to move freely is crucial for many aspects of daily life.

• The cervical spine is essential in defending the spinal cord, the bundle of neurons that carries messages from the brain to the rest of the body. The spinal cord is protected by the vertebrae and other structures in the back.

- Foramina in the cervical spine allow nerve roots to leave the spinal cord and travel to the rest of the body. Muscle contractions, sensory input, and homeostatic balance are all under the direction of the nervous system.

- The cervical spine, like the rest of the spine, contributes to good posture and balance. The health of your cervical spine depends on its proper position.

- The cervical spine also creates a passageway for the arteries and veins that transport blood to the brain. The health of the blood vessels in the brain depends on the cervical spine being properly aligned and functioning.

The shape and function of the cervical spine are crucial for many aspects of daily life, including supporting the head, aiding motions, and safeguarding the central nervous system. The health of the entire body can be maintained with proper care and attention to the cervical spine.

CHAPTER TWO
The Degenerative Nature of Cervical Spondylosis

Degenerative changes in the cervical spine cause cervical spondylosis and its many symptoms. The cervical spine and discs, as well as other neck tissues, undergo alterations during the degenerative process. Degeneration in cervical spondylosis can be summarized as follows:

- **Disc height reduction:** Degeneration typically manifests itself first in the cervical intervertebral discs. These discs dry out and become less elastic as people get older. Disc height and the discs' ability to absorb shock may both diminish as a result of dehydration.

• Bone spurs can form when the discs between the cervical vertebrae deteriorate and the vertebrae begin to rub against each other. Bony outgrowths called osteophytes or bone spurs might occur due to the increased friction. Vertebral spurs can form along the spine's periphery or inside the foramina (where nerve roots emerge from the spinal column).

• Ligaments in the cervical region may thicken and become less flexible as a result of the alterations in the spine. As a result, the neck may become more rigid and less flexible.

• The spinal canal can become constricted when disc degeneration and bone spur development work together. Spinal stenosis refers to a narrowing of the spinal canal that can irritate the spinal cord and nerve roots.

• **Compression of Nerve Roots:** Bone spurs and herniated discs can compress the nerve roots as they exit the spinal cord. Arm and hand symptoms such as tingling, numbness, and weakness may result from this pressure.

• Degenerative alterations in the cervical spine are associated with inflammation and pain in the surrounding tissues. The inflammation and the resulting mechanical compression of the spinal cord and nerves can lead to discomfort in the neck and even headaches.

• Spinal Alignment Changes Cervical degeneration, as it develops, can alter spinal alignment. Posture and equilibrium may be impacted by these alterations.

• Cervical spondylosis symptoms, such as neck stiffness and soreness, might reduce a person's ability to tilt their head and participate in specific activities.

Cervical spondylosis deterioration is a normal part of the aging process, and not everyone will develop the condition to the same extent or have the same symptoms. Symptoms can range in intensity from minor discomfort to severe pain and neurological difficulties. Symptom relief, enhanced neck function, and alleviation of problems such nerve and spinal cord compression are usual goals of treatment for cervical spondylosis. Physical therapy, pain medication, and behavioral adjustments are examples of conservative therapies. It may be essential to perform surgery to release pressure on the spinal cord or nerves.

Cervical spondylosis: Identifying the Signs

Cervical spondylosis is a degenerative disorder of the cervical spine, and its symptoms must be recognized. Cervical spondylosis may be present if any of the following occur, albeit the severity of symptoms varies from person to person:

- Cervical spondylosis is characterized by neck pain, either constant or intermittent. The discomfort or pain could be anywhere in the neck, from the base to the sides to the back.

- Cervical spondylosis patients frequently complain of neck stiffness that makes it difficult to freely turn the head or move the neck.

- Pain in the neck often spreads to the shoulders, upper back, arms, and even the hands. Compression of nerves in the neck is a common cause of this.

• Sensations of numbness, tingling, or "pins and needles" in the arms, hands, and fingers may be a symptom of cervical spondylosis. Compression of a nerve is often to blame in these cases.

• **Muscle Weakness:** If the nerves in your arms or hands are being compressed, you may experience a weakness in those muscles. This deficiency might lead to trouble with tasks that require fine motor abilities.

• Some persons with cervical spondylosis complain of headaches, which can be traced back to strained neck muscles or nerve irritation.

• Loss of Balance: Cervical spondylosis has been shown to negatively impact balance and coordination, making it more difficult to stand or walk upright.

• Dysphagia, or trouble swallowing, can occur rarely when cervical spondylosis causes compression of the esophagus.

• Rarely, but in extreme circumstances, when the spinal cord is severely compressed, people may lose control of their bladder or bowels. This is a very dangerous symptom that needs to be checked out right away.

Note that the intensity of symptoms can vary greatly, and that not everyone with cervical spondylosis will have all these symptoms. Degenerative alterations in the cervical spine might occur in some people without any obvious signs or symptoms. It is crucial to get a professional medical evaluation and diagnosis if you or someone you know is experiencing neck discomfort or related symptoms, especially if there is radiating pain, weakness, or loss of bladder or bowel control. When symptoms are identified and treated promptly, patients experience less pain and risk fewer problems.

Several illnesses and issues have been linked to cervical spondylosis and its potential for complication. The degree of these links and complications varies. Some frequent side effects of living with cervical spondylosis include:

• Compression of the spinal cord can occur as cervical spondylosis worsens and the spinal canal narrows (a condition known as spinal stenosis). Symptoms of cervical myelopathy include weakness in the arms and hands, a loss of balance, and an inability to walk.

- **Radiculopathy:** Nerve compression in the cervical spine can lead to radiculopathy. Arm and hand pain, numbness, tingling, and weakness are all symptoms of this illness. Where the nerves are compressed has a direct effect on which ones are affected.

- When cervical spondylosis causes the compression of a nerve root as it leaves the spinal cord, it can produce pain and sensory abnormalities in the area supplied by that nerve, as well as other symptoms.

• Weakness in the Arms and Hands Cervical spondylosis, by compressing nerves, can cause weakness in the arms and hands. There may be a decline in grip and fine motor skills as a result.

• **Loss of Bladder or Bowel Control (very rare):** Cervical spondylosis can cause loss of bladder or bowel control if the spinal cord is severely compressed. This is a serious health situation that needs immediate attention.

- Cervical spondylosis can induce alterations in the alignment of the cervical spine, which can manifest as a visible deformity, like a hunched forward head posture, in its more advanced stages.

- Accidental Falls and Injuries are More Likely because of Cervical Spondylosis-Related Balance and Coordination Issues.

- Because osteoarthritis is a disorder associated with age and degeneration, people with cervical spondylosis may also suffer from osteoarthritis in other joints.

- Degenerative joint disease, systemic disorders including osteoporosis, and lumbar spondylosis (degeneration of the lower back) are common companions to cervical spondylosis.

- Emotional and mental impacts include anxiety, depression, and a lower quality of life for certain people who suffer from cervical spondylosis-related chronic pain and disability.

Cervical spondylosis and its consequences and co-existing illnesses require timely diagnosis and treatment. Symptoms might be lessened and problems avoided if the condition is identified and treated early. Surgical procedures to decompress the spinal cord or nerves may be necessary in extreme situations, although non-invasive treatments such as physical therapy, pain management, anti-inflammatory drugs, and lifestyle changes are also viable possibilities. It is essential to see a doctor if you have any reason to suspect you have cervical spondylosis or are experiencing any of the associated consequences.

CHAPTER THREE
Assessment and Prognosis

Cervical spondylosis is usually diagnosed after a thorough medical history is taken, a physical examination is performed, and appropriate diagnostic tests are performed. The steps involved in identifying cervical spondylosis are as follows:

1. Health Background:

• First, your doctor will ask you a lot of questions about your health. They will inquire as to the severity, frequency, and length of your symptoms, as well as what causes or eases them.

If you have ever had neck surgery or been injured in any way, you should expect to be asked about it.

2. Health Checkup:

• Your range of motion, discomfort, and symptoms of muscular weakening or sensory abnormalities in your arms and hands are all evaluated during a physical examination of your neck.

• Problems with balance and coordination may alert the doctor to the possibility of spinal cord compression.

3. Studies in Radiology:

- Radiographs Radiographs of the cervical spine can reveal abnormalities in the bony structures, such as bone spurs, disc height alterations, and misalignment.

- When it comes to imaging soft tissues like the spinal cord, intervertebral discs, and nerve roots, nothing beats a magnetic resonance imaging (MRI) scan. Compression of the spinal cord, herniated discs, and the level of degeneration can all be revealed.

To get clear images of the cervical spine, a computed tomography (CT) scan may be prescribed. Bone density testing, detection of osteophytes (bone spurs), and detection of spinal canal narrowing are all areas where it shines.

4. Methods of Electrodiagnosis:

• Nerve function can be evaluated and damaged or compressed nerves can be located with the help of electromyography (EMG) and nerve conduction investigations. These examinations are useful for determining the extent and location of nerve problems.

5. Extra Checks:

• Cervical spondylosis can often be diagnosed with a physical exam; however, your doctor may require bloodwork to rule out other disorders that could be causing your symptoms.

6. Additional Specialized Evaluations:

• Myelography, a contrast-enhanced X-ray, and dynamic imaging (e.g., flexion-extension X-rays), are two additional procedures that may be used to assess spinal mobility and compression in a variety of contexts.

Treatment options for cervical spondylosis will be discussed with you by your doctor when a diagnosis has been made based on the evaluation and test findings. Physical therapy, anti-inflammatory medication, and lifestyle adjustments are all examples of conservative treatments that may be used. Compression of the spinal cord or a nerve may necessitate surgical intervention in extreme situations or when non-invasive therapies have failed.

Symptom relief, enhanced neck function, and slowing the disease's development are the goals of most treatments for cervical spondylosis. Depending on the intensity of symptoms and other factors, there may be a wide range of treatment options available. **Cervical spondylosis typically responds to the following treatments:**

1. Non-invasive Therapies:

• Physical therapy is commonly given to enhance the patient's neck's strength, range of motion, and posture. Physical therapists can help by providing instruction in pain management and functional restoration exercises.

- **Medications**:

Nonsteroidal anti-inflammatory medicines (NSAIDs) and other pain relievers, available without a doctor's prescription, can help lessen inflammation and discomfort.

Neck muscle spasms can be relieved with the help of muscle relaxants.

Injections of corticosteroids, which can reduce inflammation and alleviate pain, may be advised in specific circumstances.

- **Changes in Ways of Life:**

Good posture, ergonomic workspaces, and avoiding aggravating activities can all assist.

Stress on the cervical spine can be lessened with weight management.

- Physical activity, including low-impact aerobics and gentle neck exercises, can enhance neck function.

2. Soft cervical collars are sometimes recommended to alleviate pressure on the cervical spine. However, it is generally advised against using a cervical collar for an extended period of time due to the risk of muscle atrophy.

3. When applied to the affected area, heat or cold packs can alleviate pain and ease muscular tension. Some people find relief when they alternate between hot and cold applications.

4. To reduce stress and increase range of motion in the neck, manual therapies such chiropractic adjustments, osteopathic manipulation, and massage treatment may be tried.

5.Acupuncture is a supplementary therapy for cervical spondylosis that involves inserting very thin needles into particular locations on the body.

6. Nerve pain drugs like gabapentin or pregabalin may be recommended if cervical spondylosis is causing your symptoms.

7. In circumstances where non-invasive therapies have failed and severe spinal cord or nerve compression exists, surgery may be recommended. Possible surgical procedures include:

Surgery to remove a herniated disc is called a discectomy.

Stabilizing the spine by joining together two or more vertebrae is called spinal fusion.

Foraminotomy, or "nerve root opening enlargement," is a surgical procedure used to treat nerve compression.

Laminectomy refers to the surgical removal of the lamina, or back, of a vertebra in order to enlarge the spinal canal.

The responsiveness to first treatments, the intensity of symptoms, and the presence of neurological abnormalities are all important considerations when deciding on a course of treatment. The best course of treatment for your ailment will be determined in conjunction with your healthcare professional. In order to track your progress and make any necessary adjustments to your treatment plan, it is crucial that you regularly attend follow-up appointments with your healthcare professional.

CHAPTER FOUR
Cervical Spondylosis: A Daily Reality

Maintaining a high quality of life while dealing with cervical spondylosis requires treatment of the underlying condition as well as symptom management. Although cervical spondylosis is a degenerative and chronic disorder, there are ways to manage the symptoms and difficulties it causes. If you suffer from cervical spondylosis, consider the following advice:

• Comply with Your Doctor's Orders: You and your doctor should collaborate to create and stick to a specific course of treatment. This may include physical therapy, drugs, lifestyle adjustments, and, in rare situations, surgical interventions. Keeping up with your prescribed medication will help you control your symptoms and delay the onset of any further damage.

- Pain and inflammation can be managed with over-the-counter or prescribed drugs. Always with your doctor before taking any new medication, and pay attention to any warning labels.

- **Physical Therapy:** Do the exercises and stretches your

physiotherapist has given you to strengthen your neck and improve your range of motion and posture. Regular physical treatment can help alleviate discomfort and improve neck mobility.

• **Good Posture:** Keep a straight back and shoulders to reduce neck pain. To encourage proper posture while working, ergonomic adjustments like an ergonomic chair and keyboard can be made to your workspace.

• Stress on the cervical spine can be lessened with proper weight management. If you are overweight, a healthy diet and regular exercise can help you reach your goal weight and maintain it.

• Exercise on a regular basis, even if it's just walking or a stationary bike, will help keep your neck healthy and functioning properly. Activities like swimming, walking, and yoga, as well as gentle neck exercises, can help.

• Applying heat or cold packs to the neck might help alleviate pain and relax the muscles. Find the optimal temperature by trying various settings.

• **Lifestyle Modifications:** Avoid activities or positions that increase your discomfort. Reduce unnecessary stress on your neck by making the appropriate adjustments to your daily routine and workplace.

• Use a cervical collar for short-term support if your doctor advises one. However, long-term use should be avoided since it may lead to muscle weakening.

• Pain and tension can be alleviated by lowering stress levels. To better handle stress, try some deep breathing exercises, some meditation, or some attentive awareness.

• Keeping a pain diary can help you recognize trends or triggers in your pain. Your doctor may use this data to better evaluate your condition.

• **Medication Administration:** If your doctor has prescribed painkillers, be sure to take them exactly as prescribed and keep an eye out for any adverse reactions.

• **Nutrition and Diet:** Eat a healthy, anti-inflammatory diet. Antioxidants and omega-3 fatty acids are two nutrients that have shown promise in lowering inflammation and bolstering general health.

- Maintain regular contact with your doctor and let them know right away if your condition worsens or improves.

- **Surgical Intervention:** If conservative therapy are inadequate and your condition worsens, consider the potential of surgical intervention. Talk to your doctor about the potential outcomes, as well as any other options you may have.

Cervical spondylosis is a chronic condition, so be prepared to make lifestyle and treatment changes over time. Visits to the doctor on a regular basis will allow your healthcare team to keep tabs on your progress and make any necessary adjustments to your treatment plan. You can live a full life with cervical spondylosis if you take an active role in your care and make healthy decisions.

Conclusion

Many people, especially older people, suffer from cervical spondylosis, a degenerative disorder of the cervical spine. Despite the potential for a wide variety of symptoms, including neck pain and stiffness and even more serious problems including nerve compression or spinal cord compression, the condition is treatable with the right care and adaptations to one's way of living.

Important things to remember about cervical spondylosis are:

Cervical spondylosis is mostly caused by the natural aging process, with additional contributing factors including genetics, previous neck injuries, bad posture, and lifestyle choices.

Cervical spondylosis can be diagnosed using a combination of the patient's medical history, a thorough physical examination, and imaging techniques (such as X-rays or MRIs) to evaluate the cervical spine's health.

Cervical spondylosis can be treated with conservative methods such physical therapy, medication, and behavioral adjustments. When spinal cord or nerve compression becomes unbearable, surgical intervention may be necessary.

Spinal cord compression, radiculopathy, muscle weakness, and balance problems are all possible sequelae of cervical spondylosis. Loss of bowel or bladder control is possible in extremely unusual cases.

Cervical spondylosis is a degenerative neck condition that can be managed by following a treatment plan, reducing discomfort and inflammation, keeping active, and keeping excellent posture.

Keep in mind that cervical spondylosis can develop at different rates and cause varying degrees of discomfort in different people. Improving quality of life and avoiding problems depend on prompt diagnosis and treatment. Maintaining good management of cervical spondylosis requires regular contact with a healthcare provider and commitment to treatment programs. Many people with this illness can lead normal

lives with the help of appropriate
treatment strategies.

THE END